ANAPHYLAXIS

Recognizing, Treating, and Preventing Anaphylaxis: A Comprehensive Handbook

CARL JUAN

Table of Contents

Introductory

Immediately following contact with an allergen, anaphylaxis can manifest as a severe and potentially fatal allergic reaction. It's a systemic reaction that has the potential to impact multiple bodily systems, including the skin, lungs, heart, and intestines. Foods (such as peanuts and shellfish), insects (such as bees and wasps), drugs, latex, and even latex gloves can all cause anaphylaxis in some people.

Common anaphylactic symptoms include:

• Skin reactions, such as hives or swelling of the face and lips.

- Breathing problems, such as wheezing.

- The pulse is quick and feeble.

- Reduced blood pressure, resulting in lightheadedness or fainting.

- Constipation, diarrhoea, and/or nausea.

Anaphylactic shock is a potentially fatal complication of anaphylaxis in which the body's organs do not receive adequate blood flow and oxygen levels.

When someone is having an anaphylactic reaction, they need medical help immediately. In order to stop the allergic reaction and stabilize the patient, epinephrine (adrenaline) is often administered. In addition to epinephrine, antihistamines and corticosteroids may be used to treat symptoms and stop the reaction from happening again. You should always have an epinephrine auto-injector on you and know how to use it if you or someone you know has a history of severe allergies and is at risk of anaphylaxis.

CHAPTER ONE
Anaphylaxis Triggers

Different people have different sensitivities, thus it's impossible to generalize about what causes anaphylaxis. Some typical triggers for anaphylaxis are:

• Anaphylaxis is often brought on by eating certain foods. Peanuts, tree nuts (such as almonds and cashews), shellfish, fish, milk, eggs, wheat, and soy are among the most often encountered food allergies.

• Those who are allergic to the venom of certain insects may have anaphylaxis if they are stung by one of these insects. Anaphylaxis is a serious condition that can be triggered by an allergy to insect venom.

• Medication Allergies are a serious risk for those who use certain drugs. Medication such as antibiotics (e.g., penicillin), NSAIDs, and some intravenous contrast dyes used in medical imaging can all cause anaphylaxis in some people.

• Exposure to latex, such as that found in gloves, medical equipment, or balloons, is another possible trigger for anaphylaxis. But latex allergies are uncommon compared to those caused by food or insect stings.

• Some people, especially when exercise is mixed with certain foods or environmental variables, may have anaphylaxis.

• Exposure to allergens in other substances, such as latex, some metals, or certain plants, can also trigger anaphylaxis.

• Sometimes, anaphylaxis can strike with no apparent cause, a condition known as idiopathic anaphylaxis.

It's crucial to remember that the severity and frequency of anaphylactic reactions can vary widely. Avoidance of allergens and the availability of an epinephrine auto-injector can be useful in preventing or treating anaphylaxis in people who are allergic to certain substances. If you or a loved one has a history of severe allergies or anaphylaxis, it is important that you engage with your healthcare professional to create an allergy action plan. Early detection and rapid treatment with epinephrine are critical for the management of anaphylaxis.

Causes of Anaphylaxis

There is a vast variety of allergies and chemicals that can cause anaphylaxis. Common allergens that cause anaphylaxis include:

1. The ingestion of certain foods is a well-known cause of anaphylaxis. Peanuts, tree nuts (such as almonds, walnuts, and cashews), shellfish (shrimp, crab, lobster), fish, milk, eggs, wheat, soy, sesame seeds, and so on are common dietary allergies that can trigger anaphylactic reactions.

2. Insect Stings: People who are sensitive to the venom of bees, wasps, hornets, yellow jackets, and fire ants might have a severe allergic reaction to a sting from any of these insects. Allergic reactions to insect venom can be life-threatening.

3. Pharmaceutical: Anaphylaxis can be triggered by a pharmaceutical allergy. Common pharmaceutical triggers include antibiotics (e.g., penicillin and cephalosporins), non-steroidal anti-inflammatory medications (NSAIDs), muscle relaxants, and some intravenous contrast dyes used in medical imaging.

4. Exposure to latex gloves, medical devices, or other products made from natural rubber latex can cause anaphylaxis in those who are allergic to latex.

5. Exercise-induced anaphylaxis occurs when a person experiences anaphylactic symptoms after engaging in physical activity. When exercise is paired with other triggers, such as certain meals or environmental situations, anaphylaxis can become more severe.

6. In some people, anaphylaxis can be triggered by emotional or psychological stress, especially when it is combined with other triggers.

7. Some people with severe allergies have anaphylactic shock when exposed to environmental allergens such pollen, dust mites, pet dander, and mold spores.

8. Occupational Exposures: Some persons may experience anaphylaxis in response to allergens encountered in their workplace, such as latex in healthcare settings or particular chemicals.

9. Idiopathic anaphylaxis refers to the small percentage of cases in which anaphylaxis occurs for no apparent reason. Anaphylaxis of this kind is more difficult to diagnose and treat.

People with allergies or a history of anaphylaxis should collaborate closely with their healthcare professionals to pinpoint their unique triggers and create an allergy management strategy. Important steps in preventing and treating anaphylaxis include avoiding known triggers, carrying an epinephrine auto-injector, and being aware of the condition's signs and symptoms. In the event of an anaphylactic reaction, it is crucial to recognize the symptoms quickly and provide epinephrine as soon as possible.

CHAPTER TWO
Possible Dangers

There are a number of potential triggers that can bring on anaphylaxis. These factors may render persons more susceptible to severe allergic responses. Factors that often lead to anaphylactic episodes are:

• An increased risk of anaphylaxis occurs in those who already have a history of allergic reactions when exposed to their allergens, whether those allergens are foods, insects, drugs, or latex.

• A history of anaphylaxis increases a person's likelihood of experiencing another episode when exposed to the same or a similar trigger.

• **Family History:** A family history of allergies and anaphylaxis may raise the likelihood of an individual having allergies and experiencing anaphylaxis.

• Anaphylaxis can strike at any age; however it is more common in young people. Due to their immature immune systems and increased exposure to novel allergens, young children may be at a greater risk.

• People with asthma are more likely to have a life-threatening allergic reaction, such as anaphylaxis. The difficulty breathing caused by anaphylaxis might be made worse by asthma.

• An higher chance of developing allergies and, possibly, anaphylaxis, is also connected with conditions like atopic dermatitis (eczema) and allergic rhinitis (hay fever).

• A history of allergic reaction to stinging insects such as bees, wasps, and fire ants increases a person's risk of anaphylaxis if stung by one of these insects.

• The risk of anaphylaxis in reaction to different triggers may be higher in people who suffer from polyallergy, defined as an allergy or sensitivity to more than one allergen.

• Physical activity may increase the risk of exercise-induced anaphylaxis in some people, especially when paired with other risk factors like eating certain foods.

• People with latex allergies can have anaphylactic reactions if they come into contact with anything made with latex.

It's crucial for persons at risk of anaphylaxis to consult with healthcare experts to identify their unique triggers and build an allergy action plan. Strategies for avoiding allergies, recognizing the early warning signs of anaphylaxis, and, if necessary, administering epinephrine, may all be part of this action plan. Those who are at high risk for anaphylaxis should always have an epinephrine auto-injector on them in case they experience a severe allergic response.

Symptoms and Indicators

Anaphylaxis is a potentially fatal allergic reaction that requires immediate medical attention. Anaphylaxis symptoms can appear quickly, usually within minutes to an hour after being exposed to an allergen. These signs and symptoms can affect different body systems and can range in intensity depending on the affected individual. Anaphylaxis often manifests with the following signs and symptoms:

1. Sensitive Skin:

• A rash that spreads over the body (urticaria) or hives.

Angioedema, which causes swelling of the throat, lips, and tongue.

• Skin irritation/redness.

2. Breathing problems, such as feeling short of breath.

• Breathing that is labored or very loud.

To cough.

• Chest pain or tightness.

• A hoarse voice.

3. Signs of Cardiovascular Disease:

• Rapid or erratic heartbeat.

The result of a dramatic drop in blood pressure is:

Sensation of vertigo.

Syncope, or passing out.

Consciousness Dissipation.

4. Diarrhea and/or nausea.

· Stomach aches and cramps.

A case of diarrhea.

5. Extra Symptoms:

• Anxiety, dread, or a sense of impending calamity.

• A state of mind where reasoning is impaired.

Weakness; exhaustion.

• Pallor (pale skin).

It's crucial to keep in mind that not every case of anaphylaxis will exhibit all of these symptoms, and that the severity of symptoms might vary widely. Without immediate medical attention, anaphylaxis can rapidly escalate into a potentially fatal state known as anaphylactic shock.

It is crucial to respond quickly if you notice the following signs of anaphylaxis in yourself or someone else:

• When accessible and prescribed, epinephrine should be administered.

• Please dial 911 or get immediate medical attention.

• Maintain blood flow by lying down or sitting with your legs slightly elevated.

• Keep your cool; getting worked up will only make things worse.

• Follow the directions on your epinephrine auto-injector and use it if you experience a severe allergic reaction while you wait for medical assistance.

In order to effectively treat anaphylaxis, it is essential that medical professionals recognize the symptoms quickly. Epinephrine can save lives by halting an allergic reaction. After getting emergency medical care, patients experiencing anaphylaxis may require ongoing treatment and surveillance to ensure that the reaction does not repeat.

CHAPTER THREE
Anaphylaxis Diagnosis

Clinical evaluation, medical history, and the identification of symptoms and signs are often used together to make a diagnosis of anaphylaxis. An anaphylactic reaction can be identified in the following ways:

• When a patient arrives with symptoms and signs that may indicate anaphylaxis, a medical professional will conduct a complete clinical evaluation. Checking the patient's pulse, respiration rate, and oxygen saturation levels are all part of this process.

• Diagnosing anaphylaxis requires a thorough investigation of the patient's medical background. The healthcare provider will inquire as to whether or not the patient has been exposed to any known allergens or triggers. Previous allergic responses will be investigated, especially those that need immediate medical attention.

• Examine the patient's skin for signs of anaphylaxis such hives and swelling, listen for wheezing and check for other changes in vital signs to determine the severity of the patient's condition.

- The allergens that cause anaphylactic responses can be pinpointed using allergy testing. Blood testing (that look for allergen-specific IgE antibodies) and skin prick tests are two common methods. These checks might help verify suspicions of an allergy to a specific chemical.

- Care Providers May Rule Out Other Possible Diagnosis Such as Asthma Exacerbations, Cardiovascular Events, and Less Severe Allergic Reactions The healthcare practitioner may rule out other disorders that could present with similar symptoms.

• Established diagnostic criteria, such as those established by the National Institute of Allergy and Infectious Diseases (NIAID) and the Food Allergy and Anaphylaxis Network (FAAN), can be used by healthcare providers to help with a diagnosis.

• The presence of sudden, severe symptoms affecting the skin, mucosa, or both (e.g., hives, edema, or flushing), combined with respiratory symptoms and/or a drop in blood pressure.

Quick onset of symptoms, typically within minutes to hours of contact with a suspected allergen.

At least two of the following organ systems are involved: the skin, the respiratory system, the cardiovascular system, the digestive system, or the central nervous system.

• The patient's reaction to treatment is one of the most crucial indicators of a correct diagnosis. Improvement in symptoms after administration of epinephrine is diagnostic of anaphylaxis.

• Medical records should include information about the patient's illness and any identified triggers or allergens in order to better direct therapy and prevent further exposures.

Anaphylaxis diagnosis is essentially a clinical process based on the above mentioned criteria. Treatment with epinephrine should begin immediately, not wait for a diagnosis, because early recognition and treatment are crucial to improving results. Seek quick medical assistance and use an epinephrine auto-injector if one has been prescribed if you suspect anaphylaxis or encounter severe allergic reactions.

Curbing Allergy Attacks

Those at risk for anaphylaxis should take precautions to prevent potential triggers and train for emergency responses. Important measures to avoid anaphylaxis include:

• Knowing what substances can cause anaphylactic reactions in you or a loved one is essential if you or they have a history of allergies or anaphylaxis. If you think you might have an allergy, talk to your doctor about getting tested.

• Once you know what triggers your allergies, you can take preventative measures to limit your contact with the offending substances. Some examples include being aware of the potential for cross-contamination in the kitchen and advising restaurants and food service providers of any food sensitivities you may have.

• Consider donning a medical alert necklace or bracelet that lists your food allergies and/or anaphylaxis risk. This might be especially crucial in emergency situations when you may not be able to communicate.

• If you have been instructed to carry an epinephrine auto-injector (such an EpiPen), keep it on you at all times. You and the people closest to you should be proficient in its utilization. Get a new one before it runs out.

• Make a Plan for Handling Allergies
You and your doctor should create a strategy for handling your allergies. An anaphylactic action plan will include what to do in the event of an allergic reaction, including how to recognize the symptoms and when to administer an epinephrine auto-injector. Talk about it with your loved ones and your helpers.

• Make sure the people around you are aware of your sensitivities and what to do if an emergency arises. Everyone you know counts, from relatives to classmates to bosses.

• Be Cautious with Medications If you have any preexisting sensitivities to medicines, be sure to tell your doctor before getting any prescriptions or undergoing any medical procedures. Over-the-counter drugs may include allergies, so read labels carefully.

• Stinging Insect Allergies: If you have a history of allergic responses to insect stings, take precautions when outside, especially during warm months. Put on protective gear, don't use perfume, and take measures to avoid getting stung by insects.

• If you have a latex allergy, tell your doctor, dentist, and employer so that you can be certain of working in a latex-free environment.

• Those who suffer from exercise-induced anaphylaxis need to be very careful about how their workouts and meals overlap, and they may want to consider working out with someone who is also aware of their condition.

• Pollen, dust mites, and pet dander are all examples of environmental allergens that should be avoided if they induce symptoms. In addition to taking prescription allergy medicine, you may need to use an air purifier and make your environment less allergenic.

• Schedule regular checkups with your doctor so that you can be closely monitored and can discuss any changes to your allergy profile.

Anaphylaxis can be avoided with the right amount of awareness, planning, and management of allergies and recognized triggers. If you think you're having an anaphylactic response, get medical help right away and follow the instructions on your epinephrine auto-injector. Early intervention is crucial in controlling anaphylaxis.

CHAPTER FOUR
Treatment of Anaphylaxis

Prevention, symptom detection, and rapid treatment are the three pillars of anaphylaxis management. Here is a detailed plan for handling anaphylaxis:

1. Prevention:

• Figure out what you're allergic to and how to avoid it, and tell people about your condition.

If you're supposed to have an epinephrine auto-injector on you, don't forget to keep it fresh.

• Let people know about your sensitivities by donning medical alert jewelry.

2. Understanding the Signs:

• Anaphylaxis symptoms can range from mild skin reactions (hives, swelling) to life-threatening respiratory distress and cardiovascular problems, so it's important to be aware of them.

• Symptoms can occur swiftly, frequently within minutes to an hour following contact to an allergen.

3. Be prompt:

• Do not wait if you or someone with you is experiencing anaphylactic symptoms. Time is of the essence.

• If an epinephrine auto-injector has been prescribed and is available, use it immediately. Use the auto-injector in accordance with the manufacturer's instructions.

• Immediately dial 911 or get to a hospital if you need medical attention. Medical examination is still necessary after epinephrine has been given.

4. Positioning:

• Lie down or sit with your legs elevated (if feasible). The likelihood of passing out can be decreased and blood flow increased in this way.

5. Don't Panic:

• Maintain as much composure as you can. Worry and stress just make things worse.

6. Epinephrine Injection Number Two

• If symptoms persist or worsen after the initial dose of epinephrine, it may be necessary to administer a second injection. If your doctor or allergy action plan calls for a second dose, be sure to take it as directed.

7. Assistive Therapy:

•	Antihistamines and corticosteroids may be prescribed by emergency medical technicians to assist alleviate symptoms.

Blood pressure can be maintained and oxygen levels maintained with the help of intravenous (IV) fluids and possibly other treatments.

8. Observation:

• You may be watched for a few hours after the initial treatment to check for any signs of delayed or returning symptoms.

9. Follow-Up:

• It's crucial to schedule a follow-up appointment with your doctor after experiencing an anaphylactic reaction so that you can be evaluated further, talk about your triggers, and make any required changes to your allergy action plan.

10. Future Reaction Prevention:

• Consult with medical professionals to narrow down potential allergens and triggers, then make a plan to avoid them in the future.

11. Education:

• Family, friends, instructors, and coworkers are just some of the people who should know about your allergies and what to do if an allergic reaction occurs.

To save your life or the life of someone you care about, you must be ready to act quickly in the event of anaphylaxis. Rapid injection of epinephrine is the cornerstone of anaphylaxis management, with further medical attention provided for any lingering symptoms. In the case of an anaphylactic reaction, being prepared with an epinephrine auto-injector and an allergy action plan can make a world of difference.

Managing Worry and Panic

Coping with fear and worry, especially in the context of a severe allergic reaction or anaphylaxis, can be tough. Some methods for dealing with these feelings are listed below.

1. Knowledge and Learning:

• If you know what causes your anxiety, you can take steps to alleviate it. The signs of anaphylaxis and how to administer an epinephrine auto-injector are both something you should educate yourself on. When you have the facts, you can make decisions that are in your best interest.

2. Get Expert Advice:

• Talking to a mental health expert like a therapist or counselor can be helpful if anxiety and fear are severely interfering with your everyday life.

3. Methods of Deep Relaxation and Breathing:

• Anxiety can be alleviated with practices such as deep breathing, meditation, and gradual muscle relaxation. Practice these tactics regularly to build resilience to stress.

4. Practices of Mindfulness and Rooting:

• Practicing mindfulness can help you focus on the here-and-now and lessen worries about the future. Focus your mind again with the "5-4-3-2-1" technique or another grounding exercise.

5. Backing Structures:

• Share your worries and concerns with those you care about. They are able to provide comfort and sympathy. Talking about your problems with someone else can help you feel less isolated.

6. Therapy or Peer Support:

• Join a group for people who suffer from allergies or anaphylaxis. It can be comforting to talk to other people who share your worries and hear how they overcame their problems.

7. Medication that is Appropriate:

• To help their patients cope with anxiety, doctors sometimes prescribe antidepressants or anti-anxiety drugs. If you have concerns, you should talk to your doctor about this.

8. Exercising on a Regular Basis:

• Exercising can help ease stress and boost happiness levels. Endorphins, which are produced during regular exercise, are known to improve mood.

9. Nutrition and Diet:

• Pay attention to your diet and nutrition. Caffeine and sugar are both linked to increased anxiety, so limiting your intake may help. Maintain a healthy state of mind by eating right.

10. Methods of Distraction:

• Do things that make you happy and take your mind off your worries. Distracting oneself with a hobby, a book, some music, or a movie might help the mind take a break.

11. Gradual Inoculation:

• The anxiety-inducing stimulus can be faced gradually in order to desensitize the individual to it. If exposure therapy seems like it could help, talk to your therapist about creating a plan.

12. Organize and get ready:

• Knowing what to do in the event of an allergic response will help ease your mind. Keep an epinephrine auto-injector and an allergy action plan handy at all times.

13. Practice encouraging internal dialogue:

• Interrupt irrational and destructive thoughts by substituting more positive and logical ones. Remind yourself of your capacity to handle your health and stay safe.

Anxiety is a normal response to a potentially life-threatening circumstance, but it is important to remember that it is also manageable. Try to be kind with yourself and get assistance if you feel stuck. You can learn to manage your anxiety and worry about anaphylaxis and allergies with time and the correct resources.

Concerns Related to Children

Children have specific demands and potential obstacles that must be taken into account when managing anaphylaxis. Here are some things to keep in mind when dealing with anaphylaxis in children:

• Allergy testing is helpful for kids who have a family history of severe allergies. The development of a management strategy is greatly aided by the identification of specific allergies. Skin prick testing or blood tests for allergen-specific IgE antibodies can help detect triggers.

• A child's caregivers (parents, guardians, teachers, and school staff) should also be trained about anaphylaxis. Teach the child to recognize their symptoms and the necessity of immediately reporting any signs of an allergic reaction.

• Create a detailed plan for handling the child's allergies in conjunction with the doctor. When an allergic reaction occurs, this strategy should outline when and how to deliver epinephrine using an auto-injector. Talk about this strategy with your child's teachers and parents.

• Make sure the child's epinephrine auto-injectors are easily accessible at school and anywhere else he or she spends time. Talk to the school administration about where and how to keep epinephrine.

• Educators, school nurses, and administrators should all be kept in the loop on your progress and any concerns you may have as a student. Discuss the child's allergies and the allergy action plan, and make sure everyone is informed of the child's condition.

• If your kid has food allergies, talk to the school about creating a plan for managing these allergies in the classroom and cafeteria. Make sure labels are read and food is not contaminated.

• Raise awareness among the child's peers about the child's food allergies and the significance of not sharing food or possibly allergic things, as appropriate for the child's age. This can help establish a friendly atmosphere.

• As children get older, they should be taught how to take care of themselves, including how to use an epinephrine auto-injector to treat an allergic reaction. They need to have maturity level abilities and understanding.

• When talking to a child about allergies or anaphylaxis, it's important to keep in mind the child's age and use language and concepts that are age-appropriate. The child may feel less anxious and more in command of the situation.

• It's important to teach kids to detect their own symptoms, like itching, hives, swelling, or abdominal pain. Let them know how important it is to report symptoms right away.

• Plan playdates and other activities around the child's allergy action plan, and make sure other caregivers know about the child's illness and the plan.

• Special Considerations for Teenagers: Adolescents with allergies may be at heightened risk due to a desire for independence. Remind them to bring their epinephrine auto-injector and to make smart decisions about what to eat when they go out to a restaurant with their pals.

• Schedule follow-up sessions with the child's healthcare professional to check on their progress, make any necessary changes to the allergy action plan, and address any worries you may have.

When dealing with a child who has anaphylaxis, it's important for everyone involved (doctors, parents, teachers) to work together. To keep kids safe and make sure they can live healthy, active lives despite their allergies, education, awareness, and good communication are crucial.

Conclusion

When exposed to allergens or triggers, some people may experience anaphylaxis, a severe and potentially fatal allergic reaction. Symptoms might manifest on the skin, respiratory tract, cardiovascular system, or digestive system, and commonly occur together. Effective management of anaphylaxis requires rapid recognition and treatment.

Some important facts to keep in mind with anaphylaxis are:

• Foods, insect stings, medicines, latex, and other allergies are only some of the many potential causes of anaphylaxis.

• It is crucial to engage with healthcare specialists to identify specific triggers and build an allergy action plan.

• Epinephrine is the first line of defense in treating anaphylaxis, and prompt medical assistance is essential.

Those at risk for anaphylaxis and their caregivers should always have epinephrine auto-injectors on hand.

• Avoiding triggers, spreading awareness, and stocking up on supplies are all important preventative measures for treating anaphylaxis.

• Education, support, and methods to minimize stress and anxiety may be helpful for coping with fear and anxiety related to anaphylaxis.

• Special care, including education, communication, and age-appropriate talks, is required when dealing with anaphylaxis in children.

While anaphylaxis is a potentially fatal medical condition, it is manageable and the risk of anaphylactic reactions can be reduced with education, planning, and support for those affected.

THE END